ULTIMATE USMLE STEP 1 PREP

100 Essential Questions for
International Medical Graduates

Essam Abdelhakim

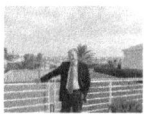

Copyright © 2024 Essam Abdelhakim

All rights reserved

The characters and events portrayed in this book are fictitious. Any similarity to real persons, living or dead, is coincidental and not intended by the author.

No part of this book may be reproduced, or stored in a retrieval system, or transmitted in any form or by any means, electronic, mechanical, photocopying, recording, or otherwise, without express written permission of the publisher.

Cover design by: Art Painter
Library of Congress Control Number: 2018675309
Printed in the United States of America

CONTENTS

Title Page
Copyright
Introduction
Questions&answers   1
Matching Questions   60
About The Author   67
DIsclosure   69

INTRODUCTION

The USMLE Step 1 exam assesses your understanding and ability to apply important concepts of the sciences basic to the practice of medicine, with a focus on principles and mechanisms underlying health, disease, and modes of therapy.

This book offers a curated collection of 100 matching questions and multiple-choice questions (MCQs) that reflect the style and difficulty of those you will encounter on the actual exam.

Each question is followed by a detailed explanation to help you understand the reasoning behind the correct answer, reinforcing your learning and ensuring you grasp the key concepts.

The questions cover a broad range of topics essential for the USMLE Step 1, including biochemistry, genetics, pharmacology, pathology, microbiology, physiology, and clinical medicine.

QUESTIONS&ANSWERS

Q1:A 50-Year-Old Man With A History Of Myocardial Infarction Is Prescribed A Medication That Selectively Blocks Beta-1 Adrenergic Receptors. Which Of The Following Cardiovascular Parameters Is Most Likely Affected By This Medication?

A. Heart rate

B. Systemic vascular resistance

C. Total peripheral resistance

D. Renal blood flow

E. Cardiac contractility

Answer: A. Heart rate

Explanation: Beta-1 adrenergic receptors are primarily located in the heart. Blocking these receptors decreases heart rate (negative chronotropic effect) as well as cardiac contractility (negative inotropic effect).

Q2:A 35-Year-Old Woman Presents With A Painful Genital Ulcer. She Reports Multiple Sexual Partners And Inconsistent Condom Use. A Smear Of The Ulcer Base Reveals Intracellular Donovan Bodies Within Mononuclear Cells. Which Of The Following Is The Most Likely Causative Organism?

A. Treponema pallidum

B. Chlamydia trachomatis

C. Haemophilus ducreyi

D. Herpes simplex virus (HSV)

E. Gardnerella vaginalis

Answer: C. Haemophilus ducreyi

Explanation: Haemophilus ducreyi causes chancroid, a sexually transmitted infection characterized by painful genital ulcers with a base containing intracellular Donovan bodies.

Q3:A 60-Year-Old Man Presents With A History Of Recurrent Kidney Stones. Laboratory Tests Reveal Elevated Serum Calcium And Parathyroid Hormone (Pth) Levels. Which Of The Following Is The Most Likely Cause Of His Hypercalcemia?

A. Hyperparathyroidism

B. Hypoparathyroidism

C. Vitamin D deficiency

D. Renal failure

E. Hyperthyroidism

Answer: A. Hyperparathyroidism

Explanation: Hyperparathyroidism leads to excessive PTH secretion, which increases bone resorption and renal calcium reabsorption, resulting in hypercalcemia.

Q4:A 25-Year-Old Woman Is Diagnosed With

A Condition Characterized By Café-Au-Lait Spots, Axillary Freckling, Lisch Nodules, And Neurofibromas. Which Of The Following Genes Is Most Likely Mutated In This Condition?

A. NF1

B. APC

C. BRCA1

D. RET

E. PTEN

Answer: A. NF1

Explanation: Neurofibromatosis type 1 (NF1) is caused by mutations in the NF1 gene, which regulates cell growth. Clinical features include café-au-lait spots, axillary freckling, Lisch nodules (iris hamartomas), and neurofibromas.

Q5:A 40-Year-Old Man Presents With A Sudden Onset Of Severe Chest Pain Radiating To His Back. He Is Diaphoretic And Hypertensive. An Electrocardiogram (Ecg) Shows St-Segment Elevation In Leads V1 To V4. Which Of The Following Is The Most Likely Diagnosis?

A. Acute pericarditis

B. Acute myocardial infarction (AMI)

C. Aortic dissection

D. Pulmonary embolism

E. Esophageal spasm

Answer: C. Aortic dissection

Explanation: Aortic dissection typically presents with severe chest pain radiating to the back, diaphoresis, and hypertension. ECG may show nonspecific changes, but ST-segment elevation in leads V1 to V4 can occur due to myocardial ischemia from coronary involvement.

Q6: A 50-Year-Old Woman With Chronic Knee Pain Undergoes An Imaging Study That Reveals Joint Space Narrowing, Osteophyte Formation, And Subchondral Sclerosis. Which Of The Following Is The Most Likely Diagnosis?

A. Rheumatoid arthritis

B. Gout

C. Osteoarthritis

D. Psoriatic arthritis

E. Systemic lupus erythematosus (SLE)

Answer: C. Osteoarthritis

Explanation: Osteoarthritis is characterized by joint space narrowing, osteophyte formation (bone spurs), and subchondral sclerosis on imaging. It typically affects weight-bearing joints like the knees and hips.

Q7: A 30-Year-Old Man Presents With Recurrent Infections And Is Found To Have Absent Circulating B Cells Due To A Genetic Defect Affecting B Cell Maturation In The Bone Marrow. Which Of The Following Is The Most Likely Diagnosis?

A. Common variable immunodeficiency (CVID)

B. X-linked agammaglobulinemia (XLA)

C. DiGeorge syndrome

D. Hyper-IgM syndrome

E. Ataxia-telangiectasia

Answer: B. X-linked agammaglobulinemia (XLA)

Explanation: XLA is caused by a mutation in the BTK gene, leading to a block in B cell maturation and absent B cells in the peripheral blood, resulting in recurrent bacterial infections due to lack of antibody production.

Q8: A 65-Year-Old Woman With Osteoporosis Is Prescribed A Medication That Inhibits Osteoclastic Bone Resorption By Binding To Hydroxyapatite Crystals In Bone. This Medication Primarily Acts By Which Of The Following Mechanisms?

A. Decreasing osteoblastic activity

B. Inhibiting vitamin D metabolism

C. Increasing intestinal calcium absorption

D. Promoting osteoclastic apoptosis

E. Decreasing osteoclastic activity

Answer: E. Decreasing osteoclastic activity

Explanation: Bisphosphonates (e.g., alendronate) inhibit osteoclastic bone resorption by binding to hydroxyapatite crystals, leading to decreased osteoclast activity and bone turnover.

Q9: A 22-Year-Old Woman Presents With Fever, Headache, And A Maculopapular Rash That Started On Her Face And Spread To Her Trunk And Extremities. She Reports Recent Travel To Central America. Which Of The Following Is The Most Likely Causative Organism?

A. Dengue virus

B. Zika virus

C. Chikungunya virus

D. Measles virus

E. Rubella virus

Answer: C. Chikungunya virus

Explanation: Chikungunya virus infection presents with fever, severe arthralgia, and a maculopapular rash starting on the face and spreading to the trunk and extremities. It is transmitted by Aedes mosquitoes and is endemic in Central America.

Q10: A 30-Year-Old Man Presents With Confusion And Muscle Weakness. Laboratory Tests Reveal Severe Hypoglycemia. He Responds Well To Intravenous Glucose Infusion. Which Of The Following Enzymes Is Most Likely Deficient In This Patient?

A. Glucokinase

B. Glucose-6-phosphatase

C. Phosphofructokinase

D. Fructose-1,6-bisphosphatase

E. Pyruvate carboxylase

Answer: B. Glucose-6-phosphatase

Explanation: Deficiency of glucose-6-phosphatase impairs gluconeogenesis and glycogenolysis, leading to hypoglycemia due to the inability to release glucose from glycogen stores or generate glucose from non-carbohydrate precursors.

Q11: A 30-Year-Old Woman Presents With Dysuria And Urinary Frequency. Urinalysis Shows Pyuria And Bacteriuria. Culture Reveals Colonies That Are Lactose Fermenting And Pink On Macconkey Agar. Which Of The Following Is The Most Likely Causative Organism?

A. Escherichia coli

B. Enterococcus faecalis

C. Klebsiella pneumoniae

D. Proteus mirabilis

E. Pseudomonas aeruginosa

Answer: A. Escherichia coli

Explanation: Escherichia coli is the most common cause of uncomplicated urinary tract infections (UTIs), characterized by pyuria and bacteriuria. It ferments lactose and appears pink on MacConkey agar.

Q12: A 55-Year-Old Woman Presents With Tingling

Sensations In Her Hands And Feet. Laboratory Tests Reveal Low Serum Vitamin B12 Levels And Elevated Methylmalonic Acid And Homocysteine Levels. Which Of The Following Is The Most Likely Cause Of Her Condition?

A. Pernicious anemia

B. Iron deficiency anemia

C. Folate deficiency

D. Chronic kidney disease

E. Thiamine deficiency

Answer: A. Pernicious anemia

Explanation: Pernicious anemia results from autoimmune destruction of gastric parietal cells, leading to vitamin B12 deficiency. Elevated methylmalonic acid and homocysteine levels are characteristic biochemical findings.

Q13: A 45-Year-Old Man Presents With Sudden-Onset Severe Abdominal Pain That Radiates To His Back. On Physical Examination, He Is Diaphoretic And Tachycardic. Abdominal Ct Scan Reveals A Retroperitoneal Hematoma. Which Of The Following Is The Most Likely Diagnosis?

A. Acute pancreatitis

B. Acute cholecystitis

C. Acute mesenteric ischemia

D. Abdominal aortic aneurysm (AAA) rupture

E. Acute appendicitis

Answer: D. Abdominal aortic aneurysm (AAA) rupture

Explanation: AAA rupture presents with sudden-onset severe abdominal or back pain, often with hypotension, diaphoresis, and a pulsatile abdominal mass. Retroperitoneal hematoma on imaging is characteristic.

Q14: A 50-Year-Old Woman Presents With Chronic Cough And Hemoptysis. Chest X-Ray Shows A Solitary Pulmonary Nodule With Irregular Borders. Biopsy Reveals Small, Round, Blue Cells With Scant Cytoplasm And Nuclear Molding. Which Of The Following Is The Most Likely Diagnosis?

A. Adenocarcinoma

B. Squamous cell carcinoma

C. Small cell lung carcinoma

D. Bronchial carcinoid tumor

E. Metastatic melanoma

Answer: C. Small cell lung carcinoma

Explanation: Small cell lung carcinoma is characterized by small, round, blue cells with scant cytoplasm and nuclear molding on histology. It typically presents as a central lung mass and is associated with paraneoplastic syndromes.

Q15: A 25-Year-Old Woman Presents With Recurrent Respiratory Tract Infections Since Childhood. Laboratory Tests Reveal Absent Cd40 Ligand Expression On T Cells. Which Of The Following Is

The Most Likely Diagnosis?

A. Hyper-IgM syndrome

B. Common variable immunodeficiency (CVID)

C. X-linked agammaglobulinemia (XLA)

D. DiGeorge syndrome

E. Ataxia-telangiectasia

Answer: A. Hyper-IgM syndrome

Explanation: Hyper-IgM syndrome is characterized by defective class switching in B cells due to mutations in CD40 ligand gene (CD40LG), leading to recurrent infections and normal or elevated IgM levels with low IgG and IgA levels.

Q16: A 65-Year-Old Man With Chronic Obstructive Pulmonary Disease (Copd) Is Prescribed A Medication That Antagonizes Muscarinic Acetylcholine Receptors In The Airways. This Medication Primarily Acts By Which Of The Following Mechanisms?

A. Relaxing bronchial smooth muscle

B. Inhibiting mast cell degranulation

C. Reducing inflammatory cytokine production

D. Increasing surfactant production

E. Inhibiting leukotriene synthesis

Answer: A. Relaxing bronchial smooth muscle

Explanation: Antimuscarinic drugs (e.g., ipratropium, tiotropium) block muscarinic receptors in the airways, leading to bronchodilation by inhibiting the action of acetylcholine on smooth muscle cells.

Q17:A 30-Year-Old Man Presents With Fever, Headache, And Photophobia. Lumbar Puncture Reveals Increased White Blood Cells And Protein In The Cerebrospinal Fluid (Csf), With A Decreased Glucose Concentration. Gram Stain Of Csf Shows Gram-Negative Diplococci. Which Of The Following Is The Most Likely Causative Organism?

A. Neisseria meningitidis

B. Streptococcus pneumoniae

C. Haemophilus influenzae

D. Listeria monocytogenes

E. Cryptococcus neoformans

Answer: A. Neisseria meningitidis

Explanation: Neisseria meningitidis is a gram-negative diplococcus that commonly causes bacterial meningitis in young adults, characterized by fever, headache, photophobia, and CSF findings of increased white blood cells, protein, and decreased glucose.

Q18:A 40-Year-Old Man Presents With Persistent Joint Pain And Swelling. Laboratory Tests Reveal Elevated Serum Uric Acid Levels. Synovial Fluid Analysis Shows Needle-Shaped Crystals With

Negative Birefringence Under Polarized Light Microscopy. Which Of The Following Is The Most Likely Diagnosis?

A. Rheumatoid arthritis

B. Gout

C. Osteoarthritis

D. Pseudogout

E. Systemic lupus erythematosus (SLE)

Answer: B. Gout

Explanation: Gout is characterized by elevated serum uric acid levels and deposition of monosodium urate crystals in joints, causing acute inflammatory arthritis. Crystals appear as needle-shaped with negative birefringence under polarized light microscopy.

Q19: A 50-Year-Old Man With A History Of Type 2 Diabetes Mellitus Presents With Progressive Numbness And Tingling In His Feet. Examination Reveals Decreased Achilles Tendon Reflexes And Decreased Sensation To Light Touch And Pinprick In A Stocking-Glove Distribution. Which Of The Following Pathophysiological Mechanisms Is Most Likely Contributing To His Symptoms?

A. Autoimmune destruction of peripheral nerves

B. Segmental demyelination of peripheral nerves

C. Axonal degeneration of peripheral nerves

D. Ectopic firing of peripheral nerve fibers

E. Impaired central nervous system processing of sensory information

Answer: C. Axonal degeneration of peripheral nerves

Explanation: Diabetic peripheral neuropathy is characterized by axonal degeneration of peripheral nerves due to chronic hyperglycemia, leading to sensory deficits, decreased reflexes, and pain or numbness in a stocking-glove distribution.

Q20: A 35-Year-Old Pregnant Woman Presents For Routine Prenatal Care. Ultrasound At 18 Weeks Gestation Shows Absence Of Renal Parenchyma With Dilated Renal Pelvis And Ureters. Which Of The Following Congenital Abnormalities Is Most Likely Present In The Fetus?

A. Horseshoe kidney

B. Multicystic dysplastic kidney

C. Autosomal dominant polycystic kidney disease (ADPKD)

D. Renal agenesis

E. Potter sequence

Answer: D. Renal agenesis

Explanation: Renal agenesis is characterized by absence of one or both kidneys due to failure of kidney development during embryogenesis. It can be unilateral (one kidney absent) or bilateral (both kidneys absent).

Q21:A 25-Year-Old Man Presents With A Painful Ulcer On His Genitals. He Reports Multiple Sexual Partners And Inconsistent Condom Use. He Is Concerned About The Possibility Of Acquiring Hiv. Which Of The Following Strategies Is Most Effective In Reducing His Risk Of Acquiring Hiv Infection?

A. Routine use of barrier contraceptives

B. Abstinence from sexual activity

C. Partner reduction

D. Pre-exposure prophylaxis (PrEP) with antiretroviral therapy

E. Vaccination against HIV

Answer: D. Pre-exposure prophylaxis (PrEP) with antiretroviral therapy

Explanation: Pre-exposure prophylaxis (PrEP) with antiretroviral therapy (e.g., tenofovir/emtricitabine) is highly effective in reducing the risk of HIV transmission in individuals at high risk of infection, such as those with multiple sexual partners and inconsistent condom use.

Q22:A 30-Year-Old Woman Presents With Excessive Worry And Fear About A Wide Range Of Situations. She Often Experiences Physical Symptoms Such As Palpitations, Sweating, And Trembling.

These Symptoms Significantly Impair Her Daily Functioning. Which Of The Following Is The Most Likely Diagnosis?

A. Panic disorder

B. Generalized anxiety disorder (GAD)

C. Social anxiety disorder

D. Obsessive-compulsive disorder (OCD)

E. Post-traumatic stress disorder (PTSD)

Answer: B. Generalized anxiety disorder (GAD)

Explanation: Generalized anxiety disorder (GAD) is characterized by excessive worry and anxiety about multiple events or activities, accompanied by physical symptoms such as restlessness, fatigue, difficulty concentrating, irritability, muscle tension, and sleep disturbances.

Q23: A 50-Year-Old Woman Presents With Generalized Weakness, Muscle Cramps, And Constipation. Laboratory Tests Reveal Hypocalcemia And Elevated Serum Phosphate Levels. Which Of The Following Hormones Is Primarily Responsible For Her Electrolyte Abnormalities?

A. Parathyroid hormone (PTH)

B. Thyroid-stimulating hormone (TSH)

C. Cortisol

D. Aldosterone

E. Antidiuretic hormone (ADH)

Answer: A. Parathyroid hormone (PTH)

Explanation: Hypocalcemia and hyperphosphatemia with low PTH levels suggest hypoparathyroidism, where decreased PTH secretion leads to decreased calcium absorption from bones and kidneys, and increased phosphate reabsorption, resulting in electrolyte abnormalities.

Q24: A 45-Year-Old Man Presents With Fatigue, Pale Skin, And Shortness Of Breath On Exertion. Laboratory Tests Reveal Microcytic, Hypochromic Anemia. Iron Studies Show Decreased Serum Iron, Increased Total Iron-Binding Capacity (Tibc), And Decreased Ferritin Levels. Which Of The Following Is The Most Likely Diagnosis?

A. Iron deficiency anemia

B. Anemia of chronic disease

C. Thalassemia trait

D. Sideroblastic anemia

E. Lead poisoning

Answer: A. Iron deficiency anemia

Explanation: Iron deficiency anemia is characterized by microcytic, hypochromic red blood cells due to inadequate iron supply for hemoglobin synthesis. Iron studies show decreased serum iron, increased TIBC, and decreased ferritin levels.

Q25: A 60-Year-Old Man Presents With Gradual Onset Of Cognitive Decline, Memory Impairment, And Difficulty With Language And Problem-Solving Tasks. Neurological Examination Reveals Bilateral Cortical Atrophy On Mri. Which Of The Following Is The Most Likely Underlying Pathology?

A. Neurofibrillary tangles

B. Amyloid plaques

C. Lewy bodies

D. Pick bodies

E. Neuritic plaques

Answer: E. Neuritic plaques

Explanation: Neuritic plaques, composed of beta-amyloid protein, are characteristic pathological findings in Alzheimer's disease, contributing to cognitive decline and neuronal dysfunction seen on MRI as cortical atrophy.

Q26: A 70-Year-Old Man With A History Of Smoking Presents With Hemoptysis And Weight Loss. Chest X-Ray Reveals A Peripheral Lung Mass. Biopsy Of The Mass Shows Glandular Structures Lined By

Columnar Cells With Nuclear Pleomorphism And Hyperchromasia. Which Of The Following Is The Most Likely Diagnosis?

A. Adenocarcinoma

B. Squamous cell carcinoma

C. Small cell lung carcinoma

D. Bronchial carcinoid tumor

E. Metastatic adenocarcinoma

Answer: A. Adenocarcinoma

Explanation: Adenocarcinoma is a type of non-small cell lung carcinoma that arises from glandular structures in the lung periphery. Histologically, it is characterized by glandular structures lined by columnar cells with nuclear pleomorphism and hyperchromasia.

Q27: A 45-Year-Old Man With Hypertension Is Prescribed A Medication That Inhibits Voltage-Gated Calcium Channels In Vascular Smooth Muscle Cells. This Medication Primarily Acts By Which Of The Following Mechanisms?

A. Decreasing heart rate

B. Increasing cardiac contractility

C. Relaxing vascular smooth muscle

D. Inhibiting renin release

E. Blocking alpha-adrenergic receptors

Answer: C. Relaxing vascular smooth muscle

Explanation: Calcium channel blockers (e.g., amlodipine, nifedipine) inhibit voltage-gated calcium channels in vascular smooth muscle cells, leading to vasodilation and decreased peripheral vascular resistance.

Q28: A 25-Year-Old Woman Presents With Fever, Headache, And A Maculopapular Rash That Started On Her Wrists And Ankles And Spread Centrally. She Reports Recent Camping And Hiking Trips. Which Of The Following Is The Most Likely Causative Organism?

A. Rickettsia rickettsii

B. Borrelia burgdorferi

C. Ehrlichia chaffeensis

D. Francisella tularensis

E. Yersinia pestis

Answer: B. Borrelia burgdorferi

Explanation: Borrelia burgdorferi is the causative organism of Lyme disease, transmitted by Ixodes ticks. It presents with erythema migrans (bull's-eye rash) that starts peripherally and spreads centrally, along with flu-like symptoms.

Q29: A 50-Year-Old Man Presents With Muscle Weakness, Fatigue, And Constipation. Laboratory Tests Show Hypokalemia, Metabolic Alkalosis, And Low Urinary Calcium Excretion. Which Of

The Following Is The Most Likely Cause Of His Electrolyte Abnormalities?

A. Hyperaldosteronism

B. Hypoparathyroidism

C. Renal tubular acidosis (RTA)

D. Cushing syndrome

E. Addison disease

Answer: A. Hyperaldosteronism

Explanation: Hyperaldosteronism leads to increased renal sodium reabsorption and potassium excretion, causing hypokalemia and metabolic alkalosis. It also enhances calcium excretion, contributing to low urinary calcium levels.

Q30: A 30-Year-Old Woman Presents With Developmental Delay, Distinctive Facial Features (Including A Prominent Forehead, Large Ears, And A Long Face), Macroorchidism, And Behavioral Problems Such As Hand-Flapping And Repetitive Movements. Which Of The Following Is The Most Likely Diagnosis?

A. Fragile X syndrome

B. Down syndrome

C. Turner syndrome

D. Klinefelter syndrome

E. Prader-Willi syndrome

Answer: A. Fragile X syndrome

Explanation: Fragile X syndrome is an X-linked dominant disorder caused by a CGG trinucleotide repeat expansion in the FMR1 gene, leading to intellectual disability, distinctive facial features, macroorchidism, and behavioral abnormalities.

Q31: A 55-Year-Old Man Presents With Progressive Dyspnea On Exertion And Dry Cough. Physical Examination Reveals Digital Clubbing And Fine End-Inspiratory Crackles At The Lung Bases. Pulmonary Function Tests Show Restrictive Lung Disease Pattern With Reduced Diffusion Capacity. Which Of The Following Is The Most Likely Diagnosis?

A. Idiopathic pulmonary fibrosis (IPF)

B. Chronic obstructive pulmonary disease (COPD)

C. Sarcoidosis

D. Bronchiectasis

E. Pneumothorax

Answer: A. Idiopathic pulmonary fibrosis (IPF)

Explanation: IPF presents with progressive dyspnea, dry cough, digital clubbing, fine end-inspiratory crackles (Velcro crackles), restrictive lung disease pattern on pulmonary function tests, and reduced diffusion capacity.

Q32: A 40-Year-Old Woman Presents With Chronic Back Pain And Morning Stiffness That Improves With Activity. X-Ray Of The Sacroiliac Joints Shows Bilateral Asymmetric Sacroiliitis With Erosions And Sclerosis. Which Of The Following Is The Most Likely Diagnosis?

A. Ankylosing spondylitis

B. Osteoarthritis

C. Rheumatoid arthritis

D. Psoriatic arthritis

E. Systemic lupus erythematosus (SLE)

Answer: A. Ankylosing spondylitis

Explanation: Ankylosing spondylitis is a seronegative spondyloarthropathy characterized by bilateral asymmetric sacroiliitis on imaging, axial involvement with bamboo spine appearance, and extra-articular manifestations like uveitis.

Q33: A 20-Year-Old Woman Presents With Recurrent Respiratory Tract Infections Since Childhood. Laboratory Tests Show Absent B Cells In Peripheral Blood. Flow Cytometry Analysis Reveals A Lack Of Expression Of Cd19 And Cd20 On B Cells. Which Of The Following Is The Most Likely Diagnosis?

A. X-linked agammaglobulinemia (XLA)

B. Common variable immunodeficiency (CVID)

C. Hyper-IgM syndrome

D. Severe combined immunodeficiency (SCID)

E. Ataxia-telangiectasia

Answer: A. X-linked agammaglobulinemia (XLA)

Explanation: XLA is caused by a mutation in the BTK gene, leading to absent B cells in peripheral blood and a lack of expression of CD19 and CD20. Patients present with recurrent bacterial infections due to absent antibody production.

Q34: A 28-Year-Old Man Presents With Fever, Chills, And Severe Headache. Lumbar Puncture Reveals Cloudy Cerebrospinal Fluid (Csf) With Increased White Blood Cells, Elevated Protein, And Decreased Glucose Levels. Gram Stain Of Csf Shows Gram-Positive Cocci In Chains. Which Of The Following Is The Most Likely Causative Organism?

A. Streptococcus pneumoniae

B. Neisseria meningitidis

C. Haemophilus influenzae

D. Listeria monocytogenes

E. Staphylococcus aureus

Answer: A. Streptococcus pneumoniae

Explanation: Streptococcus pneumoniae is a common cause of bacterial meningitis in adults, presenting with acute onset of fever, headache, and altered mental status. CSF findings include increased white blood cells, elevated protein, and decreased glucose levels.

Q35: A 35-Year-Old Woman Presents With Muscle Weakness And Fatigue. Laboratory Tests Show Hypokalemia, Metabolic Alkalosis, And Elevated Serum Aldosterone Levels. Which Of The Following Conditions Is Most Likely Causing Her Symptoms?

A. Conn syndrome

B. Cushing syndrome

C. Addison disease

D. Primary hyperparathyroidism

E. Diabetes insipidus

Answer: A. Conn syndrome

Explanation: Conn syndrome (primary hyperaldosteronism) leads to excess aldosterone secretion by adrenal adenoma or hyperplasia, causing increased renal sodium reabsorption, potassium excretion, hypokalemia, and metabolic alkalosis.

Q36: A 30-Year-Old Pregnant Woman Presents For Routine Prenatal Care. Ultrasound At 20 Weeks Gestation Shows Absence Of Kidneys And Oligohydramnios. Which Of The Following Congenital Abnormalities Is Most Likely Present In The Fetus?

A. Bilateral renal agenesis

B. Autosomal dominant polycystic kidney disease (ADPKD)

C. Multicystic dysplastic kidney

D. Horseshoe kidney

E. Renal dysplasia

Answer: A. Bilateral renal agenesis

Explanation: Bilateral renal agenesis is characterized by absence of both kidneys due to failure of kidney development during embryogenesis, leading to oligohydramnios and Potter sequence.

Q37: A 25-Year-Old Man Presents With A Painless Genital Ulcer And Inguinal Lymphadenopathy. Dark-Field Microscopy Of Ulcer Exudate Shows Spirochetes. Which Of The Following Is The Most Appropriate Initial Treatment For This Patient?

A. Penicillin G benzathine

B. Acyclovir

C. Metronidazole

D. Ceftriaxone

E. Doxycycline

Answer: A. Penicillin G benzathine

Explanation: Penicillin G benzathine is the treatment of choice for primary and secondary syphilis caused by Treponema pallidum. It is given as a single intramuscular dose.

Q38: A 35-Year-Old Man Presents With Excessive Worry And Fear About A Wide Range Of Situations. He Often Experiences Physical Symptoms Such As Palpitations, Sweating, And Trembling. These Symptoms Significantly Impair His Daily Functioning. Which Of The Following Is The Most Likely Diagnosis?

A. Panic disorder

B. Generalized anxiety disorder (GAD)

C. Social anxiety disorder

D. Obsessive-compulsive disorder (OCD)

E. Post-traumatic stress disorder (PTSD)

Answer: A. Panic disorder

Explanation: Panic disorder is characterized by recurrent panic attacks with intense fear and discomfort, accompanied by physical symptoms such as palpitations, sweating, trembling, and chest pain. It causes significant impairment in daily life.

Q39: A 40-Year-Old Man Presents With Chronic Back Pain And Morning Stiffness That Improves With Activity. Laboratory Tests Show Elevated Erythrocyte Sedimentation Rate (Esr) And C-Reactive Protein (Crp) Levels. Which Of The Following Cellular Processes Is Most Likely Contributing To His Symptoms?

A. Increased osteoclastic activity

B. Decreased osteoblastic activity

C. Autoimmune destruction of joint synovium

D. Chronic inflammation of joint cartilage

E. Degeneration of joint ligaments

Answer: A. Increased osteoclastic activity

Explanation: Ankylosing spondylitis is characterized by chronic inflammation of the spine and sacroiliac joints, leading to increased osteoclastic activity and subsequent bone resorption, causing pain and stiffness worsened by rest and improved by activity.

Q40: A 35-Year-Old Woman Is Found To Have A 15Q11-13 Deletion On Chromosome Analysis. She Exhibits Moderate Intellectual Disability, Seizures, And A History Of Hyperphagia Leading To Obesity. Which Of The Following Is The Most Likely Diagnosis?

A. Prader-Willi syndrome

B. Angelman syndrome

C. Rett syndrome

D. Fragile X syndrome

E. Turner syndrome

Answer: A. Prader-Willi syndrome

Explanation: Prader-Willi syndrome results from paternal deletion or uniparental disomy of chromosome 15q11-13, causing intellectual disability, hyperphagia leading to obesity, hypogonadism, and characteristic facial features.

Q41: A 50-Year-Old Man Presents With Sudden-Onset Severe Chest Pain That Radiates To His Back. He Is Diaphoretic And Appears Anxious. Blood Pressure Is 180/110 Mmhg, Heart Rate Is 100/Min, And Respiratory Rate Is 20/Min. Ecg Shows St-Segment Elevation In Leads Ii, Iii, And Avf. Which Of The Following Is The Most Appropriate Next Step In Management?

A. Intravenous nitroglycerin

B. Coronary angiography

C. Morphine sulfate

D. Aspirin

E. Beta-blocker therapy

Answer: D. Aspirin

Explanation: This patient's presentation is consistent with acute inferior myocardial infarction. Immediate administration of aspirin (to inhibit platelet aggregation) is crucial in the management of acute coronary syndrome.

Q42: A 55-Year-Old Woman With A History Of Type 2 Diabetes Mellitus Presents With Sudden-Onset Severe Pain And Swelling In Her Right Foot. Physical Examination Reveals Erythema, Warmth, And Tenderness Over The Dorsal Aspect Of The Foot. Laboratory Tests Show Elevated Serum Uric Acid Levels. Which Of The Following Mechanisms Is Most Likely Responsible For Her Symptoms?

A. Deposition of urate crystals in joints

B. Autoimmune destruction of joint cartilage

C. Activation of osteoclasts leading to bone resorption

D. Chronic inflammation of synovial membranes

E. Degeneration of joint ligaments

Answer: A. Deposition of urate crystals in joints

Explanation: This patient's presentation is consistent with acute gouty arthritis, caused by deposition of monosodium urate crystals in joints due to hyperuricemia. It typically affects the first metatarsophalangeal joint (podagra) and presents with sudden-onset severe pain, erythema, and swelling.

Q43: A 40-Year-Old Woman Presents With Recurrent Episodes Of Headache, Visual Disturbances, And Excessive Thirst And Urination. Laboratory Tests Show Hypernatremia And Elevated Urine Osmolality Despite Dehydration. Mri Of The Sella

Turcica Reveals A Pituitary Mass Compressing Adjacent Structures. Which Of The Following Is The Most Likely Diagnosis?

A. Prolactinoma

B. Craniopharyngioma

C. Meningioma

D. Glioblastoma multiforme

E. Pituitary adenoma

Answer: E. Pituitary adenoma

Explanation: Pituitary adenomas can cause hypersecretion of hormones (e.g., growth hormone, prolactin) leading to various clinical manifestations, including headaches, visual disturbances, and diabetes insipidus due to compression of adjacent structures.

Q44: A 30-Year-Old Man Presents With Muscle Weakness, Fatigue, And Bone Pain. Laboratory Tests Show Hypophosphatemia, Hypercalcemia, And Elevated Serum Alkaline Phosphatase Levels. Serum Parathyroid Hormone (Pth) Levels Are Low. Which Of The Following Is The Most Likely Cause Of His Electrolyte Abnormalities?

A. Hyperparathyroidism

B. Vitamin D deficiency

C. Osteoporosis

D. Renal tubular acidosis (RTA)

E. Paget disease of bone

Answer: B. Vitamin D deficiency

Explanation: Vitamin D deficiency leads to impaired intestinal calcium absorption and secondary hyperparathyroidism, causing bone resorption (elevated alkaline phosphatase) and release of calcium from bones into the blood (hypercalcemia) with compensatory hypophosphatemia.

Q45: A 25-Year-Old Man Presents With Developmental Delay, Intellectual Disability, And A History Of Seizures Since Childhood. Physical Examination Reveals Macrocephaly, Coarse Facial Features, Large Tongue, And Hepatosplenomegaly. Which Of The Following Is The Most Likely Inheritance Pattern For His Condition?

A. Autosomal dominant

B. Autosomal recessive

C. X-linked recessive

D. X-linked dominant

E. Mitochondrial

Answer: C. X-linked recessive

Explanation: Hunter syndrome (Mucopolysaccharidosis type II) is an X-linked recessive disorder caused by deficiency of iduronate-2-sulfatase enzyme, leading to accumulation of glycosaminoglycans. It predominantly affects males due to X-linked recessive inheritance.

Q46: A 65-Year-Old Woman With Osteoporosis Is Prescribed A Medication That Acts As A Selective Estrogen Receptor Modulator (Serm).

This Medication Primarily Acts By Which Of The Following Mechanisms?

A. Increasing bone resorption

B. Reducing intestinal calcium absorption

C. Inhibiting osteoclastic activity

D. Enhancing parathyroid hormone (PTH) secretion

E. Blocking vitamin D receptor

Answer: C. Inhibiting osteoclastic activity

Explanation: Selective estrogen receptor modulators (e.g., raloxifene) act as estrogen agonists on bone tissue, inhibiting osteoclastic activity and reducing bone resorption, thereby preventing osteoporosis.

Q47: A 55-Year-Old Woman With A History Of Hypertension And Type 2 Diabetes Mellitus Presents With Left-Sided Weakness And Facial Droop. Ct Scan Of The Head Shows A Hyperdense Middle Cerebral Artery (Mca) Sign. Which Of The Following Is The Most Appropriate Initial Management?

A. Intravenous tissue plasminogen activator (tPA)

B. Aspirin

C. Warfarin

D. Intravenous heparin

E. Carotid endarterectomy

Answer: A. Intravenous tissue plasminogen activator (tPA)

Explanation: This patient presents with symptoms suggestive of acute ischemic stroke, and the presence of hyperdense MCA sign on CT scan suggests large vessel occlusion. Intravenous tPA is indicated within 4.5 hours of symptom onset to improve outcomes by restoring blood flow.

Q48: A 60-Year-Old Man With A History Of Hypertension And Smoking Presents With Abrupt Onset Of Severe Chest Pain That Radiates To His Back. Blood Pressure Is 180/100 Mmhg, Heart Rate Is 90/Min, And Respiratory Rate Is 22/Min. Physical Examination Reveals Diminished Left Radial Pulse And Blood Pressure Discrepancy Between Arms. Which Of The Following Is The Most Likely Underlying Pathology?

A. Aortic dissection

B. Myocardial infarction

C. Stable angina

D. Pericarditis

E. Pulmonary embolism

Answer: A. Aortic dissection

Explanation: Aortic dissection presents with sudden-onset severe chest pain that radiates to the back, hypertension with blood pressure discrepancy between arms, and pulse deficits. It requires urgent diagnosis and management to prevent complications such as aortic rupture.

Q49: A 65-Year-Old Woman With A History Of Atrial Fibrillation Presents With Severe Abdominal Pain. A Ct Angiogram Reveals A Thrombus In The

Superior Mesenteric Artery. She Is Started On An Anticoagulant. Which Of The Following Medications Is Most Likely Prescribed To Prevent Further Thromboembolism?

A. Aspirin
B. Warfarin
C. Clopidogrel
D. Heparin
E. Apixaban

Answer: E. Apixaban

Explanation: Apixaban is a direct factor Xa inhibitor used for the prevention and treatment of thromboembolic events in patients with atrial fibrillation. It is preferred over warfarin due to fewer dietary restrictions, no need for regular monitoring, and a better safety profile regarding bleeding risks.

Q50: A 30-Year-Old Woman Is Prescribed An Oral Contraceptive Pill (Ocp) Containing Ethinyl Estradiol And Norethindrone. Which Of The Following Mechanisms Primarily Accounts For The Contraceptive Effect Of This Medication?

A. Inhibition of FSH and LH secretion
B. Increase in cervical mucus viscosity
C. Acceleration of ovum transport through fallopian tubes
D. Stimulation of endometrial proliferation
E. Suppression of androgen production

Answer: A. Inhibition of FSH and LH secretion

Explanation: Oral contraceptive pills containing estrogen and progestin work primarily by inhibiting the secretion of follicle-stimulating hormone (FSH) and luteinizing hormone (LH) from the pituitary gland, thereby preventing ovulation.

Q51: A 50-Year-Old Man With Chronic Obstructive Pulmonary Disease (Copd) Is Prescribed A Long-Acting Beta-2 Agonist. Which Of The Following Medications Is Most Appropriate For This Patient?

A. Albuterol
B. Ipratropium
C. Salmeterol
D. Montelukast
E. Fluticasone

Answer: C. Salmeterol

Explanation: Salmeterol is a long-acting beta-2 agonist (LABA) used for the maintenance treatment of COPD. It helps to relax bronchial smooth muscle, providing prolonged bronchodilation. Albuterol is a short-acting beta-2 agonist, ipratropium is a short-acting anticholinergic, montelukast is a leukotriene receptor antagonist, and fluticasone is an inhaled corticosteroid.

Q52: A 45-Year-Old Man With Hypertension Is Started On An Ace Inhibitor. Which Of The Following Is The Most Likely Adverse Effect He Should Be Monitored For?

A. Bradycardia
B. Hypokalemia
C. Cough

D. Constipation
E. Hyperglycemia

Answer: C. Cough

Explanation: ACE inhibitors, such as lisinopril, can cause a persistent dry cough due to the accumulation of bradykinin. Other common side effects include hyperkalemia and angioedema. Bradycardia, constipation, and hyperglycemia are not typically associated with ACE inhibitors.

Q53: A 38-Year-Old Woman With A History Of Generalized Anxiety Disorder Is Prescribed A Medication That Enhances The Effects Of Gamma-Aminobutyric Acid (Gaba) At The Gaba-A Receptor. Which Of The Following Medications Was Most Likely Prescribed?

A. Sertraline
B. Buspirone
C. Alprazolam
D. Venlafaxine
E. Bupropion

Answer: C. Alprazolam

Explanation: Alprazolam is a benzodiazepine that enhances the effects of GABA at the GABA-A receptor, providing anxiolytic effects. Sertraline and venlafaxine are antidepressants, buspirone is an anxiolytic with a different mechanism of action, and bupropion is an atypical antidepressant.

Q54: A 70-Year-Old Man With Parkinson's Disease

Is Prescribed A Combination Of Carbidopa And Levodopa. What Is The Primary Purpose Of Adding Carbidopa To Levodopa Therapy?

A. To decrease the risk of tardive dyskinesia
B. To inhibit the peripheral conversion of levodopa to dopamine
C. To enhance the absorption of levodopa in the gastrointestinal tract
D. To provide neuroprotective effects
E. To antagonize dopamine receptors in the CNS

Answer: B. To inhibit the peripheral conversion of levodopa to dopamine

Explanation: Carbidopa is added to levodopa to inhibit dopa decarboxylase in the peripheral tissues, thereby preventing the conversion of levodopa to dopamine outside the central nervous system. This increases the availability of levodopa to cross the blood-brain barrier, where it is then converted to dopamine, and reduces peripheral side effects such as nausea and vomiting.

Q55: A 50-Year-Old Man Presents With A Chronic Cough And Hemoptysis. He Has A 30-Pack-Year Smoking History. A Chest X-Ray Reveals A Mass In The Right Upper Lobe. A Biopsy Of The Mass Shows Keratin Pearls And Intercellular Bridges. Which Of The Following Is The Most Likely Diagnosis?

A. Small cell carcinoma
B. Adenocarcinoma
C. Squamous cell carcinoma
D. Large cell carcinoma
E. Carcinoid tumor

Answer: C. Squamous cell carcinoma

Explanation: Squamous cell carcinoma of the lung is strongly associated with smoking and is characterized histologically by the presence of keratin pearls and intercellular bridges. It typically arises in the central part of the lung (hilar region) and can cause symptoms like cough and hemoptysis.

Q56: A 65-Year-Old Woman Presents With Jaundice, Pruritus, And Dark Urine. Laboratory Tests Show Elevated Bilirubin And Alkaline Phosphatase Levels. A Liver Biopsy Reveals Fibrous Obliteration Of Small Bile Ducts With Concentric "Onion Skin" Fibrosis. Which Of The Following Conditions Is Most Likely?

A. Primary sclerosing cholangitis
B. Primary biliary cirrhosis
C. Hepatitis C
D. Alcoholic cirrhosis
E. Wilson's disease

Answer: A. Primary sclerosing cholangitis

Explanation: Primary sclerosing cholangitis (PSC) is characterized by chronic cholestasis and inflammation leading to fibrous obliteration of the bile ducts with an "onion skin" appearance. It is often associated with inflammatory bowel disease, particularly ulcerative colitis.

Q57: A 35-Year-Old Woman Presents With A Painless, Firm Breast Mass. Mammography Reveals A Well-Circumscribed, Dense Lesion. A Biopsy Shows Proliferation Of Stromal And Glandular Components Without Cellular Atypia Or Mitotic Activity. Which Of The Following Is The Most Likely Diagnosis?

A. Fibroadenoma
B. Phyllodes tumor
C. Invasive ductal carcinoma
D. Lobular carcinoma in situ
E. Fibrocystic changes

Answer: A. Fibroadenoma

Explanation: Fibroadenoma is the most common benign breast tumor in young women. It presents as a painless, firm, and mobile mass. Histologically, it shows proliferation of both stromal and glandular components without atypia or significant mitotic activity.

Q58: A 7-Year-Old Boy Presents With Hematuria And Edema. Laboratory Tests Show Proteinuria And Hypoalbuminemia. A Renal Biopsy Reveals Effacement Of Podocyte Foot Processes On Electron Microscopy But No Changes On Light Microscopy. Which Of The Following Is The Most Likely Diagnosis?

A. Focal segmental glomerulosclerosis
B. Membranous nephropathy
C. Minimal change disease
D. IgA nephropathy
E. Post-streptococcal glomerulonephritis

Answer: C. Minimal change disease

Explanation: Minimal change disease is the most common cause of nephrotic syndrome in children. It is characterized by massive proteinuria, hypoalbuminemia, and edema. Electron microscopy shows effacement of podocyte foot processes, while light microscopy appears normal.

Q59: A 60-Year-Old Man With Chronic Hepatitis B Presents With Weight Loss And Right Upper Quadrant Pain. Serum Alpha-Fetoprotein Levels Are Elevated. Imaging Reveals A Liver Mass. A Biopsy Of The Mass Shows Cells With A Trabecular Pattern And Bile Production. Which Of The Following Is The Most Likely Diagnosis?

A. Hepatocellular carcinoma
B. Cholangiocarcinoma
C. Metastatic colon cancer
D. Hemangioma
E. Hepatic adenoma

Answer: A. Hepatocellular carcinoma

Explanation: Hepatocellular carcinoma (HCC) is strongly associated with chronic hepatitis B and C infections. It presents with elevated alpha-fetoprotein levels and liver mass. Histologically, HCC shows a trabecular pattern of cells and bile production.

Q60: A 35-Year-Old Man Presents With Fever, Headache, And A Rash That Began On His Wrists And Ankles And Has Spread To His Trunk. He Recently Returned From A Camping Trip In The Southeastern United States. Which Of The Following Organisms Is Most Likely Responsible For His Symptoms?

A. Borrelia burgdorferi
B. Rickettsia rickettsii
C. Ehrlichia chaffeensis

D. Coxiella burnetii
E. Francisella tularensis

Answer: B. Rickettsia rickettsii

Explanation: Rickettsia rickettsii causes Rocky Mountain spotted fever, characterized by fever, headache, and a rash that begins on the wrists and ankles and spreads to the trunk. It is transmitted by tick bites and is common in the southeastern United States.

Q61: A 45-Year-Old Woman Presents With Chronic Cough And Weight Loss. A Chest X-Ray Reveals Cavitary Lesions In The Upper Lobes Of The Lungs. Sputum Analysis Shows Acid-Fast Bacilli. Which Of The Following Is The Most Likely Diagnosis?

A. Mycobacterium tuberculosis
B. Mycoplasma pneumoniae
C. Legionella pneumophila
D. Histoplasma capsulatum
E. Nocardia asteroides

Answer: A. Mycobacterium tuberculosis

Explanation: Mycobacterium tuberculosis is the causative agent of tuberculosis, which presents with chronic cough, weight loss, and cavitary lesions in the upper lobes of the lungs. Acid-fast bacilli in sputum confirm the diagnosis.

Q62: A 6-Year-Old Boy Presents With Fever, Sore Throat, And A Sandpaper-Like Rash. Physical Examination Reveals A Strawberry Tongue And Circumoral Pallor. Which Of The Following Organisms Is Most Likely Responsible For His Condition?

A. Streptococcus pyogenes
B. Staphylococcus aureus
C. Corynebacterium diphtheriae
D. Neisseria meningitidis
E. Haemophilus influenzae

Answer: A. Streptococcus pyogenes

Explanation: Streptococcus pyogenes causes scarlet fever, characterized by fever, sore throat, a sandpaper-like rash, strawberry tongue, and circumoral pallor. It often follows streptococcal pharyngitis and is treated with antibiotics to prevent complications.

Q63: A 32-Year-Old Man With Hiv Presents With Fever, Night Sweats, And Weight Loss. His Cd4 Count Is 45 Cells/Mm³. Sputum Culture Grows Acid-Fast Bacilli. Which Of The Following Is The Most Likely Diagnosis?

A. Mycobacterium tuberculosis
B. Mycobacterium avium complex
C. Pneumocystis jirovecii
D. Histoplasma capsulatum
E. Cryptococcus neoformans

Answer: B. Mycobacterium avium complex

Explanation: Mycobacterium avium complex (MAC) is a common cause of disseminated infection in patients with advanced HIV/AIDS (CD4 count <50 cells/mm³). It presents with fever, night sweats, and weight loss, and acid-fast bacilli in sputum culture confirm the diagnosis.

Q64: A 4-Year-Old Boy Presents With Developmental Delay, Long Face, Large Ears, And Macroorchidism.

Genetic Testing Reveals An Abnormal Expansion Of Cgg Repeats. Which Of The Following Is The Most Likely Diagnosis?

A. Huntington disease
B. Myotonic dystrophy
C. Fragile X syndrome
D. Prader-Willi syndrome
E. Angelman syndrome

Answer: C. Fragile X syndrome

Explanation: Fragile X syndrome is caused by an abnormal expansion of CGG repeats in the FMR1 gene on the X chromosome. It presents with developmental delay, intellectual disability, long face, large ears, and macroorchidism.

Q65: A 25-Year-Old Woman With A Family History Of Breast Cancer Undergoes Genetic Testing And Is Found To Have A Mutation In The Brca1 Gene. Which Of The Following Is The Function Of The Normal Brca1 Gene Product?

A. Signal transduction
B. DNA repair
C. Apoptosis regulation
D. Protein synthesis
E. Cell cycle progression

Answer: B. DNA repair

Explanation: The BRCA1 gene is a tumor suppressor gene involved in the repair of double-stranded DNA breaks. Mutations in BRCA1 increase the risk of breast and ovarian cancers due to the impaired ability to repair DNA damage.

Q66: A 30-Year-Old Man Presents With Muscle Weakness And Atrophy. His Father Had Similar Symptoms And Died At Age 40. Genetic Testing Shows A Mutation In The Dmpk Gene. Which Of The Following Trinucleotide Repeats Is Associated With This Condition?

A. CAG
B. CGG
C. GAA
D. CTG
E. CTT

Answer: D. CTG

Explanation: Myotonic dystrophy is associated with an expansion of CTG trinucleotide repeats in the DMPK gene. It presents with muscle weakness, myotonia, and various systemic manifestations. The condition shows anticipation, with symptoms worsening in successive generations.

Q67: A Newborn Is Found To Have Hypotonia, Poor Feeding, And Distinctive Facial Features. Chromosomal Analysis Reveals A Deletion On Chromosome 15 Of Paternal Origin. Which Of The Following Syndromes Is Most Likely?

A. Angelman syndrome
B. Prader-Willi syndrome
C. DiGeorge syndrome
D. Williams syndrome

E. Cri-du-chat syndrome

Answer: B. Prader-Willi syndrome

Explanation: Prader-Willi syndrome is caused by a deletion on the paternal copy of chromosome 15q11-q13. It presents with hypotonia, poor feeding in infancy, hyperphagia, obesity, intellectual disability, and distinctive facial features.

Q68: A 35-Year-Old Woman Presents With Bilateral Hearing Loss And Multiple Skin Nodules. Genetic Testing Reveals A Mutation In The Nf2 Gene. Which Of The Following Is The Most Likely Inheritance Pattern Of This Condition?

A. Autosomal dominant
B. Autosomal recessive
C. X-linked dominant
D. X-linked recessive
E. Mitochondrial inheritance

Answer: A. Autosomal dominant

Explanation: Neurofibromatosis type 2 (NF2) is an autosomal dominant disorder caused by mutations in the NF2 gene, which encodes merlin, a tumor suppressor protein. It presents with bilateral vestibular schwannomas (acoustic neuromas), hearing loss, and multiple schwannomas and meningiomas.

Q69: A Couple With A History Of Recurrent Miscarriages Undergo Genetic Counseling. Karyotyping Reveals That The Woman Has A Balanced Translocation Involving Chromosomes 13 And 14. Which Of The Following Is The Most Likely Explanation For Their Recurrent Miscarriages?

A. Uniparental disomy
B. Aneuploidy
C. Robertsonian translocation
D. Trinucleotide repeat expansion
E. Genomic imprinting

Answer: C. Robertsonian translocation

Explanation: A Robertsonian translocation involves the fusion of two acrocentric chromosomes, typically chromosomes 13 and 14. This can lead to unbalanced gametes during reproduction, resulting in aneuploidy and recurrent miscarriages or chromosomal disorders such as trisomy 13 or 21.

Q70: A 30-Year-Old Woman Runs A Marathon On A Hot Day. During The Race, Her Body Loses A Significant Amount Of Water Through Sweat. Which Of The Following Changes In Renal Physiology Is Most Likely To Occur In Response To This Dehydration?

A. Decreased renin release
B. Decreased aldosterone secretion
C. Increased ADH secretion
D. Increased glomerular filtration rate
E. Increased atrial natriuretic peptide secretion

Answer: C. Increased ADH secretion

Explanation: Dehydration leads to increased plasma osmolality, which stimulates the release of antidiuretic hormone (ADH) from the posterior pituitary. ADH increases water reabsorption in the collecting ducts of the kidneys, helping to conserve water and concentrate the urine.

Q71: A 65-Year-Old Man With Chronic Obstructive Pulmonary Disease (Copd) Has Arterial Blood Gas Results Showing Ph 7.36, Pco₂ 60 Mmhg, And Hco₃⁻ 35 Meq/L. Which Of The Following Compensatory Mechanisms Is Most Likely Occurring?

A. Respiratory acidosis with renal compensation
B. Respiratory alkalosis with renal compensation
C. Metabolic acidosis with respiratory compensation
D. Metabolic alkalosis with respiratory compensation
E. Combined respiratory and metabolic acidosis

Answer: A. Respiratory acidosis with renal compensation

Explanation: The patient has a primary respiratory acidosis (elevated PCO_2) due to COPD. The compensatory mechanism involves the kidneys increasing bicarbonate (HCO_3^-) reabsorption to buffer the excess acid, resulting in a near-normal pH.

Q72: A 24-Year-Old Man Is In A Car Accident And Suffers A Traumatic Brain Injury That Damages His Hypothalamus. Which Of The Following Physiological Processes Is Most Likely To Be Directly Affected?

A. Regulation of blood glucose levels
B. Control of voluntary muscle movements
C. Maintenance of body temperature
D. Synthesis of digestive enzymes
E. Production of red blood cells

Answer: C. Maintenance of body temperature

Explanation: The hypothalamus plays a crucial role in regulating body temperature through its thermoregulatory center. Damage to this area can impair the body's ability to maintain normal temperature homeostasis.

Q73: A 50-Year-Old Woman Has A Fasting Plasma Glucose Level Of 180 Mg/Dl. Which Of The Following Hormones Is Most Likely Elevated In Response To This Hyperglycemia?

A. Insulin
B. Glucagon
C. Cortisol
D. Epinephrine
E. Growth hormone

Answer: A. Insulin

Explanation: In response to hyperglycemia, the pancreas secretes insulin to promote glucose uptake by cells and decrease blood glucose levels. Insulin facilitates the storage of glucose as glycogen in the liver and muscle tissues.

Q74: A 28-Year-Old Man Is Undergoing A Stress Test On A Treadmill. During Exercise, Which Of The Following Changes Is Most Likely To Occur In His Skeletal Muscle Vasculature?

A. Decreased blood flow due to vasoconstriction
B. Increased blood flow due to vasodilation
C. Decreased capillary permeability
D. Increased resistance in arterioles
E. Decreased production of nitric oxide

Answer: B. Increased blood flow due to vasodilation

Explanation: During exercise, skeletal muscle blood flow increases due to vasodilation mediated by local metabolic factors such as adenosine, lactate, and nitric oxide. This process ensures adequate oxygen and nutrient delivery to the active muscles.

Q75: A 70-Year-Old Woman Is Diagnosed With Congestive Heart Failure. Which Of The Following Changes Is Most Likely To Occur In Her Cardiovascular System As A Compensatory Response?

A. Decreased sympathetic nervous system activity
B. Decreased secretion of atrial natriuretic peptide
C. Increased renin-angiotensin-aldosterone system activation
D. Increased stroke volume
E. Decreased systemic vascular resistance

Answer: C. Increased renin-angiotensin-aldosterone system activation

Explanation: In congestive heart failure, decreased cardiac output triggers the activation of the renin-angiotensin-aldosterone system (RAAS) to maintain blood pressure and tissue perfusion. This leads to increased sodium and water retention, vasoconstriction, and increased blood volume, which can exacerbate heart failure symptoms.

Q76: A 45-Year-Old Man Presents With Chest Pain That Radiates To His Left Arm And Jaw. The Pain Is Exacerbated By Exertion And Relieved By Rest. His Ecg Shows St-Segment Depression. Which Of The Following Is The Most Likely Diagnosis?

A. Acute myocardial infarction
B. Stable angina
C. Unstable angina
D. Pericarditis

E. Pulmonary embolism

Answer: B. Stable angina

Explanation: Stable angina is characterized by chest pain that occurs with exertion and is relieved by rest. ST-segment depression on an ECG indicates myocardial ischemia, which is typically reversible and relieved by rest or nitroglycerin.

Q77: A 60-Year-Old Woman With A History Of Hypertension Presents With Sudden-Onset Severe Headache, Vomiting, And Neck Stiffness. A Ct Scan Of The Head Shows Blood In The Subarachnoid Space. Which Of The Following Is The Most Likely Diagnosis?

A. Ischemic stroke
B. Subdural hematoma
C. Epidural hematoma
D. Subarachnoid hemorrhage
E. Intracerebral hemorrhage

Answer: D. Subarachnoid hemorrhage

Explanation: Subarachnoid hemorrhage presents with sudden-onset severe headache (often described as the worst headache of life), vomiting, and neck stiffness. CT scan shows blood in the subarachnoid space. It is commonly caused by the rupture of a cerebral aneurysm.

Q78: A 55-Year-Old Man With Chronic Alcohol Use Presents With Abdominal Pain, Jaundice, And Ascites. Laboratory Tests Reveal Elevated Liver Enzymes And A Prolonged Prothrombin Time. Which Of The Following Is The Most Likely

Diagnosis?

A. Hepatitis A
B. Hepatitis C
C. Alcoholic cirrhosis
D. Non-alcoholic fatty liver disease
E. Wilson's disease

Answer: C. Alcoholic cirrhosis

Explanation: Alcoholic cirrhosis is a result of chronic alcohol use leading to liver damage, fibrosis, and nodular regeneration. It presents with signs of liver failure such as jaundice, ascites, elevated liver enzymes, and a prolonged prothrombin time.

Q79: A 23-Year-Old Woman Presents With Fever, Sore Throat, And Lymphadenopathy. Her Monospot Test Is Positive. Which Of The Following Complications Is Most Commonly Associated With This Infection?

A. Acute glomerulonephritis
B. Myocarditis
C. Splenic rupture
D. Rheumatic fever
E. Hepatitis

Answer: C. Splenic rupture

Explanation: Infectious mononucleosis, caused by Epstein-Barr virus, presents with fever, sore throat, and lymphadenopathy. A positive monospot test confirms the diagnosis. One of the most serious complications of infectious mononucleosis is splenic rupture due to splenomegaly.

Q80: A 32-Year-Old Man Presents With Joint Pain,

Redness, And Swelling In The Right Knee. He Also Has A Rash On His Palms And Soles And Reports A Recent History Of Urethritis. Which Of The Following Is The Most Likely Diagnosis?

A. Osteoarthritis
B. Rheumatoid arthritis
C. Psoriatic arthritis
D. Reactive arthritis
E. Septic arthritis

Answer: D. Reactive arthritis

Explanation: Reactive arthritis, also known as Reiter's syndrome, typically presents with the triad of arthritis, urethritis, and conjunctivitis. It often follows an infection, particularly gastrointestinal or genitourinary. The characteristic rash on the palms and soles is known as keratoderma blennorrhagicum.

Q81: A 65-Year-Old Woman Presents With A Persistent Cough, Hemoptysis, And Weight Loss. She Has A 40-Pack-Year Smoking History. Chest X-Ray Reveals A Mass In The Right Upper Lobe. Which Of The Following Is The Most Likely Diagnosis?

A. Chronic bronchitis
B. Tuberculosis
C. Lung cancer
D. Pulmonary embolism
E. Pneumonia

Answer: C. Lung cancer

Explanation: Lung cancer should be highly suspected in a patient with a significant smoking history who presents with cough, hemoptysis, weight loss, and a mass on chest X-ray. The right upper lobe is a common location for lung cancer to develop.

Q82:A 35-Year-Old Woman Presents With Right Upper Quadrant Pain, Fever, And Jaundice. An Ultrasound Of The Abdomen Shows Dilated Bile Ducts And A Stone In The Common Bile Duct. Which Of The Following Is The Most Likely Diagnosis?

A. Acute cholecystitis
B. Acute pancreatitis
C. Choledocholithiasis
D. Hepatocellular carcinoma
E. Hepatitis

Answer: C. Choledocholithiasis

Explanation: Choledocholithiasis refers to the presence of a stone in the common bile duct. This condition can cause right upper quadrant pain, fever, jaundice, and dilated bile ducts on ultrasound.

Q83:A 70-Year-Old Man With A History Of Smoking Presents With Hematuria And Weight Loss. A Ct Scan Of The Abdomen Reveals A Mass In The Left Kidney. Which Of The Following Is The Most Likely Diagnosis?

A. Renal cell carcinoma
B. Polycystic kidney disease
C. Pyelonephritis
D. Nephrolithiasis
E. Hydronephrosis

Answer: A. Renal cell carcinoma

Explanation: Renal cell carcinoma is a common type of kidney cancer that often presents with hematuria, weight loss, and a mass on imaging. Risk factors include smoking and older age.

Q84: A 45-Year-Old Woman Presents With Sudden Onset Of Severe Headache, Described As The Worst Headache Of Her Life. A Non-Contrast Ct Scan Of The Head Shows Hyperdensity In The Basal Cisterns. Which Of The Following Is The Most Likely Diagnosis?

A. Subdural hematoma
B. Epidural hematoma
C. Subarachnoid hemorrhage
D. Intracerebral hemorrhage
E. Ischemic stroke

Answer: C. Subarachnoid hemorrhage

Explanation: A subarachnoid hemorrhage typically presents with a sudden, severe headache and is characterized by hyperdensity in the basal cisterns on a non-contrast CT scan. It is often caused by a ruptured aneurysm.

Q85: A 60-Year-Old Woman Presents With Progressive Difficulty Swallowing Solid Foods. A Barium Swallow Study Reveals A "Bird-Beak" Appearance Of The Distal Esophagus. Which Of The Following Is The Most Likely Diagnosis?

A. Achalasia
B. Esophageal cancer
C. Gastroesophageal reflux disease (GERD)
D. Peptic ulcer disease
E. Esophageal stricture

Answer: A. Achalasia

Explanation: Achalasia is characterized by a "bird-beak" appearance of the distal esophagus on barium swallow study, due to failure of the lower esophageal sphincter to relax and loss of esophageal peristalsis. This results in progressive dysphagia.

Q86: A 25-Year-Old Man Presents After A Motor Vehicle Accident With Chest Pain And Shortness Of Breath. A Chest X-Ray Shows Multiple Rib Fractures And A Pneumothorax On The Right Side. Which Of The Following Is The Best Next Step In Management?

A. Administering oxygen therapy
B. Performing needle decompression
C. Inserting a chest tube
D. Intubating the patient
E. Performing a thoracotomy

Answer: C. Inserting a chest tube

Explanation: In the case of a pneumothorax, especially in the setting of trauma with rib fractures, the best next step is to insert a chest tube to re-expand the lung and evacuate the air from the pleural space.

Q87: A 50-Year-Old Woman With A History Of Breast Cancer Treated With Lumpectomy And Radiation Therapy Presents With A Palpable Breast Mass. A Mammogram Shows A Spiculated Mass With Microcalcifications. Which Of The Following Is The Most Likely Diagnosis?

A. Fibroadenoma
B. Breast cyst
C. Recurrence of breast cancer
D. Fat necrosis
E. Mastitis

Answer: C. Recurrence of breast cancer

Explanation: A spiculated mass with microcalcifications on a mammogram in a patient with a history of breast cancer is highly suggestive of recurrence. The spiculated appearance and microcalcifications are characteristic features of malignancy.

Q88: A 3-Month-Old Infant Presents With Vomiting, Irritability, And Poor Feeding. Blood Tests Reveal Hypoglycemia, Lactic Acidosis, Hyperlipidemia, And Hyperuricemia. A Liver Biopsy Shows Glycogen Accumulation. Which Of The Following Enzymes Is Most Likely Deficient In This Patient?

A. Glucose-6-phosphatase
B. Glycogen phosphorylase
C. Alpha-1,4-glucosidase
D. Debranching enzyme
E. Pyruvate dehydrogenase

Answer: A. Glucose-6-phosphatase

Explanation: The patient likely has von Gierke disease (type I glycogen storage disease), caused by a deficiency of glucose-6-phosphatase. This enzyme deficiency leads to glycogen accumulation, hypoglycemia, lactic acidosis, hyperlipidemia, and hyperuricemia.

Q89: A 25-Year-Old Man Presents With Muscle

Cramps And Myoglobinuria After Intense Exercise. Blood Tests Reveal Elevated Creatine Kinase Levels. Which Of The Following Metabolic Disorders Is Most Likely Responsible For These Symptoms?

A. McArdle disease
B. Pompe disease
C. Cori disease
D. Hers disease
E. Andersen disease

Answer: A. McArdle disease

Explanation: McArdle disease (type V glycogen storage disease) is caused by a deficiency in muscle glycogen phosphorylase. It presents with exercise-induced muscle cramps, myoglobinuria, and elevated creatine kinase levels.

Q90:A 30-Year-Old Woman Presents With Fatigue, Pallor, And A Sore Tongue. Blood Tests Reveal Megaloblastic Anemia. Her Serum Homocysteine Levels Are Elevated, But Her Methylmalonic Acid Levels Are Normal. Which Of The Following Deficiencies Is Most Likely?

A. Vitamin B6 (pyridoxine)
B. Vitamin B12 (cobalamin)
C. Folate
D. Iron
E. Vitamin C (ascorbic acid)

Answer: C. Folate

Explanation: Megaloblastic anemia with elevated homocysteine and normal methylmalonic acid levels indicates a folate deficiency. Both vitamin B12 and folate deficiencies can cause megaloblastic anemia, but only vitamin B12 deficiency will also elevate methylmalonic acid levels.

Q91: A 5-Year-Old Boy Presents With Developmental Delay And A Musty Odor. Blood Tests Reveal Elevated Phenylalanine Levels. Which Of The Following Enzymes Is Most Likely Deficient In This Patient?

A. Tyrosinase
B. Homogentisate oxidase
C. Phenylalanine hydroxylase
D. Branched-chain alpha-keto acid dehydrogenase
E. Cystathionine synthase

Answer: C. Phenylalanine hydroxylase

Explanation: The patient likely has phenylketonuria (PKU), caused by a deficiency in phenylalanine hydroxylase. This enzyme deficiency leads to elevated levels of phenylalanine and its metabolites, resulting in developmental delay and a characteristic musty odor.

Q92: A 40-Year-Old Man Presents With Darkening Of The Urine When It Is Left Standing And Arthralgia. He Is Diagnosed With Alkaptonuria. Which Of The Following Metabolic Pathways Is Affected In This Condition?

A. Glycogenolysis
B. Urea cycle
C. Phenylalanine and tyrosine degradation
D. Fatty acid oxidation
E. Purine metabolism

Answer: C. Phenylalanine and tyrosine degradation

Explanation: Alkaptonuria is caused by a deficiency in homogentisate oxidase, an enzyme involved in the degradation of phenylalanine and tyrosine. This leads to the accumulation of homogentisic acid, which causes dark urine and ochronosis.

Q93: A 7-Year-Old Girl Presents With Failure To Thrive, Hepatomegaly, And Cataracts. Her Urine Tests Positive For Reducing Substances. Which Of The Following Enzyme Deficiencies Is Most Likely In This Patient?

A. Galactose-1-phosphate uridyltransferase
B. Aldolase B
C. Fructokinase
D. Galactokinase
E. Hexokinase

Answer: A. Galactose-1-phosphate uridyltransferase

Explanation: The patient likely has classic galactosemia, caused by a deficiency in galactose-1-phosphate uridyltransferase. This enzyme deficiency leads to the accumulation of galactose-1-phosphate and galactitol, resulting in hepatomegaly, cataracts, and positive urine reducing substances.

MATCHING QUESTIONS

Q94: Match The Genetic Disorder With The Corresponding Enzyme Deficiency.

1. Phenylketonuria (PKU)
2. Tay-Sachs disease
3. Gaucher disease
4. Pompe disease
5. Maple syrup urine disease

A. Hexosaminidase A
B. Glucocerebrosidase
C. Phenylalanine hydroxylase
D. Alpha-1,4-glucosidase
E. Branched-chain alpha-keto acid dehydrogenase

Answers:

1. C (Phenylalanine hydroxylase)
2. A (Hexosaminidase A)
3. B (Glucocerebrosidase)
4. D (Alpha-1,4-glucosidase)
5. E (Branched-chain alpha-keto acid dehydrogenase)

Q95: Match The Hormone With Its Primary Action.

1. Insulin
2. Glucagon
3. Cortisol

4. Parathyroid hormone (PTH)
5. Aldosterone

A. Increases blood glucose levels by promoting gluconeogenesis
B. Lowers blood glucose levels by facilitating cellular glucose uptake
C. Increases blood calcium levels by stimulating osteoclast activity
D. Increases reabsorption of sodium in the kidneys
E. Increases blood glucose levels by promoting glycogenolysis

Answers:

1. (Lowers blood glucose levels by facilitating cellular glucose uptake)
2. (Increases blood glucose levels by promoting glycogenolysis)
3. A (Increases blood glucose levels by promoting gluconeogenesis)
4. C (Increases blood calcium levels by stimulating osteoclast activity)
5. D (Increases reabsorption of sodium in the kidneys)

Q96: Match The Hypersensitivity Reaction Type With Its Description.

1. Type I (Immediate)
2. Type II (Cytotoxic)
3. Type III (Immune Complex)
4. Type IV (Delayed)

A. Mediated by IgE antibodies and mast cells, leading to anaphylaxis
B. Mediated by T cells, resulting in contact dermatitis
C. Mediated by IgG or IgM antibodies against cell surface antigens, leading to cell destruction

D. Mediated by immune complexes, leading to systemic inflammation

Answers:

1.A (Mediated by IgE antibodies and mast cells, leading to anaphylaxis)
2.C (Mediated by IgG or IgM antibodies against cell surface antigens, leading to cell destruction)
3.D (Mediated by immune complexes, leading to systemic inflammation)
4.B (Mediated by T cells, resulting in contact dermatitis)

Q97:Match The Vitamin With Its Deficiency Manifestation.

1.Vitamin A
2.Vitamin B1 (Thiamine)
3.Vitamin B12 (Cobalamin)
4.Vitamin C (Ascorbic acid)
5.Vitamin D

A. Rickets or osteomalacia
B. Night blindness and xerophthalmia
C. Scurvy
D. Beriberi or Wernicke-Korsakoff syndrome
E. Megaloblastic anemia and neurological symptoms

Answers:

1.B (Night blindness and xerophthalmia)
2.D (Beriberi or Wernicke-Korsakoff syndrome)

3.E (Megaloblastic anemia and neurological symptoms)
4.C (Scurvy)
5.A (Rickets or osteomalacia)

Q98:Match The Type Of Collagen With Its Primary Location.

1.Type I collagen
2.Type II collagen
3.Type III collagen
4.Type IV collagen

A. Basal lamina of epithelial cells
B. Hyaline cartilage
C. Bone, skin, tendon
D. Blood vessels, granulation tissue

Answers:

1.C (Bone, skin, tendon)
2.B (Hyaline cartilage)
3.D (Blood vessels, granulation tissue)
4.A (Basal lamina of epithelial cells)

Q99: Match The Pathogen With The Disease It Most Commonly Causes.

1. Mycobacterium tuberculosis
2. Treponema pallidum
3. Borrelia burgdorferi
4. Plasmodium falciparum
5. Varicella-zoster virus

A. Lyme disease
B. Syphilis
C. Tuberculosis
D. Malaria
E. Chickenpox and shingles

Answers:

1. C (Tuberculosis)
2. B (Syphilis)
3. A (Lyme disease)
4. D (Malaria)
5. E (Chickenpox and shingles)

Q100: Match The Enzyme Inhibitor With Its Effect On Enzyme Kinetics.

1. Competitive inhibitor

2. Non-competitive inhibitor
3. Uncompetitive inhibitor

A. Decreases Vmax and Km
B. Increases Km, no change in Vmax
C. Decreases Vmax, no change in Km

Answers:

1. B (Increases Km, no change in Vmax)
2. C (Decreases Vmax, no change in Km)
3. A (Decreases Vmax and Km)

ABOUT THE AUTHOR

Essam Abdelhakim

Senior consultant and Expert in Medical Education

DISCLOSURE

Disclosure

This book has been created with the assistance of *Artificial Intelligence (AI) tools* and thoroughly reviewed and edited by the author to ensure clarity, relevance, and educational value.

While every effort has been made to provide accurate and up-to-date information, this content is intended solely for educational and informational purposes.

The author is a medical professional; however, the information provided in this book *is not a substitute for professional medical advice, diagnosis, or treatment.*

Readers are strongly advised to consult licensed healthcare providers or specialists for any medical concerns or conditions.

By using this book, **you acknowledge and agree** that the author shall not be held responsible or liable for any loss, damage, or harm whether physical, emotional, financial, or otherwise that may occur *as a result of the use or misuse of the information presented herein.*

www.ingramcontent.com/pod-product-compliance
Lightning Source LLC
Chambersburg PA
CBHW071954210526
45479CB00003B/936